I0453646

Solutions For Healthy Living

Copyright © 2022 Jennifer Williams

Published by
Jennifer Williams

All rights reserved. No part of this publication may be reproduced, distributed, or transmitted in any form or by any means, including photocopying, recording, or other electronic or mechanical methods, without the prior written permission of the publisher, except in the case of brief quotations embodied in critical reviews and certain other noncommercial uses permitted by copyright law. For permission requests, write to the publisher, addressed "Attention: Permissions Coordinator," at the address below.

Email: jwilliams@Solutions-Co.com
www.Solutions-Co.com

ISBN: 979-8-218-03990-5
Audience: 13 & Up

Cover design and Interior Layout by Krystle Walton

Printed in the United States of America

Hi, I am Jennifer, a Licensed Professional Counselor, National Board-Certified Counselor and Certified Professional Counselor Supervisor.

Solutions For Healthy Living is a Self-Help, Journal- Workbook. This Journal-Workbook was created, to help individuals learn to develop better problem-solving skills. I would like to teach you how to identify, think through and potentially resolve the issue(s), by challenging your negative self-talk and cognitive distortions. Your thoughts have a direct impact on your feelings and emotions. However, if you can gain control over your thoughts by processing, exploring, and challenging the thoughts that have triggered those uncomfortable emotions, you can change the way you feel.

Additionally, this Journal-Workbook will allow you to focus on prayer, gratitude, positive affirmations, and daily goals. So often, we focus on what is going wrong and the negatives, that we often forget about the positives and small WINS!

This Journal-workbook is easy to follow. There are eight repetitive pages throughout. There are three pages that will allow you to freestyle with your journal entry, prayer and to document your gratitude. The other five pages are structured and will prompt you to read and answer questions that will challenge you do some processing and identify some healthy solutions.

This Journal-Workbook can be utilized by individuals ages 13 and older.

I hope that you find this Journal-Workbook helpful in your journey to emotional freedom and your growth and development process.

"Experience some of Life's Greatest Gifts ... PEACE and HAPPINESS"

My Prayer For Today

(This can be a personal prayer or reference a scripture)

Date: _____

_____

_____

_____

_____

_____

_____

_____

_____

_____

_____

_____

_____

_____

_____

_____

_____

Date:_____

Today's Journal Entry

_____

_____

_____

_____

_____

_____

_____

_____

_____

_____

_____

_____

_____

_____

_____

_____

_____

_____

_____

_____

Date: _____

Identify the problem:

_____

_____

_____

_____

_____

_____

Identify your thoughts and feelings related to the problem:

_____

_____

_____

_____

_____

_____

_____

_____

_____

_____

_____

How can I challenge my thoughts and feelings related to the problem?

_____

_____

_____

_____

_____

1. Is there any proof or facts that support my thoughts and feelings ? *(Only go by what you have heard verbatim from the source or seen directly.)* Have you addressed the situation to support your feelings?

Yes (Explain):_____

_____

_____

_____

No (Explain):_____

_____

_____

2. What story, scenario, and or assumptions have I created in my head?

_____

_____

_____

_____

_____

_____

_____

_____

3. After answering the previous two questions, share your new perspective, thoughts and feelings about the situation.

_____

_____

_____

_____

_____

_____

4. What is a realistic solution? Identify steps that help you move forward.

A. _____

_____

_____

B. _____

_____

_____

C. _____

_____

_____

D. _____

_____

_____

Daily Affirmations

I am:
_____

_____

_____

_____

_____

_____

_____

I will:
_____

_____

_____

_____

_____

_____

_____

I can:
_____

_____

_____

_____

_____

_____

Date: _____

Today's Goals

Today I will:

_____

_____

_____

_____

_____

_____

_____

_____

Today I will not:

_____

_____

_____

_____

_____

_____

_____

_____

What I Am Grateful For

_____

_____

_____

_____

_____

_____

_____

_____

_____

_____

_____

_____

_____

_____

_____

_____

_____

_____

My Prayer For Today

(This can be a personal prayer or reference a scripture)

Date: _____

_____

_____

_____

_____

_____

_____

_____

_____

_____

_____

_____

_____

_____

_____

_____

_____

Date:_____

Today's Journal Entry

Date: _____

Identify the problem:

_____
_____
_____
_____
_____
_____
_____

Identify your thoughts and feelings related to the problem:

_____
_____
_____
_____
_____
_____
_____
_____
_____
_____
_____

How can I challenge my thoughts and Feelings related to the problem?

_____

_____

_____

_____

1. Is there any proof or facts that support my thoughts and Feelings ? *(Only go by what you have heard verbatim from the source or seen directly.)* Have you addressed the situation to support your Feelings?

Yes (Explain): _____

_____

_____

No (Explain): _____

_____

_____

2. What story, scenario, and or assumptions have I created in my head?

_____

_____

_____

_____

_____

_____

3. After answering the previous two questions, share your new perspective, thoughts and feelings about the situation.

_____

_____

_____

_____

_____

_____

4. What is a realistic solution? Identify steps that help you move forward.

A. _____

_____

_____

B. _____

_____

_____

C. _____

_____

_____

D. _____

_____

_____

Daily Affirmations

I am:

_____

_____

_____

_____

_____

_____

_____

I will:

_____

_____

_____

_____

_____

_____

I can:

_____

_____

_____

_____

_____

Today's Goals

Today I will:

_____

_____

_____

_____

_____

_____

_____

_____

Today I will not:

_____

_____

_____

_____

_____

_____

_____

_____

What I Am Grateful For

_____

_____

_____

_____

_____

_____

_____

_____

_____

_____

_____

_____

_____

_____

_____

_____

_____

_____

_____

My Prayer For Today

(This can be a personal prayer or reference a scripture)

Date: _____

_____

_____

_____

_____

_____

_____

_____

_____

_____

_____

_____

_____

_____

_____

_____

_____

Date:_____

Today's Journal Entry

Date: _____

Identify the problem:

_____
_____
_____
_____
_____
_____
_____

Identify your thoughts and feelings related to the problem:

_____
_____
_____
_____
_____
_____
_____
_____
_____
_____
_____
_____
_____

How can I challenge my thoughts and feelings related to the problem?

Date: _____

_____

_____

_____

_____

_____

1. Is there any proof or facts that support my thoughts and feelings? *(Only go by what you have heard verbatim from the source or seen directly.)* Have you addressed the situation to support your feelings?

Yes (Explain): _____

_____

_____

No (Explain): _____

_____

_____

2. What story, scenario, and or assumptions have I created in my head?

_____

_____

_____

_____

_____

_____

_____

3. After answering the previous two questions, share your new perspective, thoughts and feelings about the situation.

_____

_____

_____

_____

_____

_____

4. What is a realistic solution? Identify steps that help you move forward.

A. _____

_____

_____

B. _____

_____

_____

C. _____

_____

_____

D. _____

_____

_____

Daily Affirmations

I am:

_____

_____

_____

_____

_____

_____

_____

I will:

_____

_____

_____

_____

_____

_____

_____

I can:

_____

_____

_____

_____

_____

_____

_____

Today's Goals

Today I will:

_____

_____

_____

_____

_____

_____

_____

_____

Today I will not:

_____

_____

_____

_____

_____

_____

_____

_____

What I Am Grateful For

_____

_____

_____

_____

_____

_____

_____

_____

_____

_____

_____

_____

_____

_____

_____

_____

_____

_____

My Prayer For Today

(This can be a personal prayer or reference a scripture)

Date: _____

_____

_____

_____

_____

_____

_____

_____

_____

_____

_____

_____

_____

_____

_____

_____

_____

Date:_____

Today's Journal Entry

Date: _____

Identity the problem:

_____

_____

_____

_____

_____

_____

_____

Identity your thoughts and feelings related to the problem:

_____

_____

_____

_____

_____

_____

_____

_____

_____

_____

_____

How can I challenge my thoughts and feelings related to the problem?

_____

_____

_____

_____

_____

1. Is there any proof or facts that support my thoughts and feelings ? *(Only go by what you have heard verbatim from the source or seen directly.)* Have you addressed the situation to support your feelings?

Yes (Explain):

_____

_____

_____

No (Explain):

_____

_____

_____

2. What story, scenario, and or assumptions have I created in my head?

_____

_____

_____

_____

_____

_____

_____

3. After answering the previous two questions, share your new perspective, thoughts and feelings about the situation.

_____

_____

_____

_____

_____

_____

4. What is a realistic solution? Identify steps that help you move forward.

A. _____

_____

_____

B. _____

_____

_____

C. _____

_____

_____

D. _____

_____

_____

Daily Affirmations

I am:
_____

_____

_____

_____

_____

_____

_____

I will:
_____

_____

_____

_____

_____

_____

I can:
_____

_____

_____

_____

_____

Today's Goals

Today I will:

_____
_____
_____
_____
_____
_____
_____
_____

Today I will not:

_____
_____
_____
_____
_____
_____
_____
_____
_____

What I Am Grateful For

_____

_____

_____

_____

_____

_____

_____

_____

_____

_____

_____

_____

_____

_____

_____

_____

_____

_____

My Prayer For Today

(This can be a personal prayer or reference a scripture)

Date: _____

_____

_____

_____

_____

_____

_____

_____

_____

_____

_____

_____

_____

_____

_____

_____

Date:_____

Today's Journal Entry

Date: _____

Identify the problem:

_____

_____

_____

_____

_____

_____

_____

Identify your thoughts and feelings related to the problem:

_____

_____

_____

_____

_____

_____

_____

_____

_____

_____

_____

How can I challenge my thoughts and feelings related to the problem?

Date: _____

_____

_____

_____

_____

1. Is there any proof or facts that support my thoughts and feelings ? *(Only go by what you have heard verbatim from the source or seen directly.)* Have you addressed the situation to support your feelings?

Yes (Explain): _____

_____

_____

No (Explain): _____

_____

_____

2. What story, scenario, and or assumptions have I created in my head?

_____

_____

_____

_____

_____

_____

_____

3. After answering the previous two questions, share your new perspective, thoughts and feelings about the situation.

_____

_____

_____

_____

_____

_____

4. What is a realistic solution? Identify steps that help you move forward.

A. _____

_____

_____

B. _____

_____

_____

C. _____

_____

_____

D. _____

_____

_____

Daily Affirmations

I am:

_____

_____

_____

_____

_____

_____

I will:

_____

_____

_____

_____

_____

I can:

_____

_____

_____

_____

Today's Goals

Today I will:

_____

_____

_____

_____

_____

_____

_____

_____

Today I will not:

_____

_____

_____

_____

_____

_____

_____

_____

What I Am Grateful For

_____

_____

_____

_____

_____

_____

_____

_____

_____

_____

_____

_____

_____

_____

_____

_____

_____

_____

My Prayer For Today

(This can be a personal prayer or reference a scripture)

Date: _____

_____

_____

_____

_____

_____

_____

_____

_____

_____

_____

_____

_____

_____

_____

_____

_____

_____

Date: _____

Today's Journal Entry

_____

_____

_____

_____

_____

_____

_____

_____

_____

_____

_____

_____

_____

_____

_____

_____

_____

_____

_____

_____

Date: _____

Identify the problem:

_____

_____

_____

_____

_____

_____

Identify your thoughts and feelings related to the problem:

_____

_____

_____

_____

_____

_____

_____

_____

_____

_____

_____

_____

How can I challenge my thoughts and feelings related to the problem?

_____

_____

_____

_____

1. Is there any proof or facts that support my thoughts and feelings ? *(Only go by what you have heard verbatim from the source or seen directly.)* Have you addressed the situation to support your feelings?

Yes (Explain): _____

_____

_____

No (Explain): _____

_____

_____

2. What story, scenario, and or assumptions have I created in my head?

_____

_____

_____

_____

_____

_____

3. After answering the previous two questions, share your new perspective, thoughts and feelings about the situation.

_____

_____

_____

_____

_____

_____

4. What is a realistic solution? Identify steps that help you move forward.

A. _____

_____

_____

B. _____

_____

_____

_____

C. _____

_____

_____

D. _____

_____

_____

Daily Affirmations

I am:

_____

_____

_____

_____

_____

_____

_____

I will:

_____

_____

_____

_____

_____

_____

I can:

_____

_____

_____

_____

_____

_____

Today's Goals

Today I will:

_____

_____

_____

_____

_____

_____

_____

_____

_____

Today I will not:

_____

_____

_____

_____

_____

_____

_____

_____

_____

What I Am Grateful For

_____

_____

_____

_____

_____

_____

_____

_____

_____

_____

_____

_____

_____

_____

_____

_____

_____

_____

_____

My Prayer For Today

(This can be a personal prayer or reference a scripture)

Date: _____

_____

_____

_____

_____

_____

_____

_____

_____

_____

_____

_____

_____

_____

_____

_____

_____

Date:_____

Today's Journal Entry

_____

_____

_____

_____

_____

_____

_____

_____

_____

_____

_____

_____

_____

_____

_____

_____

_____

_____

_____

_____

Identify the problem:

_____

_____

_____

_____

_____

_____

_____

Identify your thoughts and feelings related to the problem:

_____

_____

_____

_____

_____

_____

_____

_____

_____

_____

_____

How can I challenge my thoughts and feelings related to the problem?

_____

_____

_____

_____

1. Is there any proof or facts that support my thoughts and feelings? *(Only go by what you have heard verbatim from the source or seen directly.)* Have you addressed the situation to support your feelings?

Yes (Explain):

_____

_____

_____

No (Explain):

_____

_____

_____

2. What story, scenario, and or assumptions have I created in my head?

_____

_____

_____

_____

_____

_____

_____

3. After answering the previous two questions, share your new perspective, thoughts and feelings about the situation.

_____

_____

_____

_____

_____

_____

4. What is a realistic solution? Identify steps that help you move forward.

A. _____

_____

_____

B. _____

_____

_____

_____

C. _____

_____

_____

D. _____

_____

_____

Daily Affirmations

I am:
_____
_____
_____
_____
_____
_____
_____

I will:
_____
_____
_____
_____
_____
_____

I can:
_____
_____
_____
_____
_____

Date: _____

Today's Goals

Today I will:

_____
_____
_____
_____
_____
_____
_____
_____
_____

Today I will not:

_____
_____
_____
_____
_____
_____
_____
_____
_____
_____

What I Am Grateful For

_____

_____

_____

_____

_____

_____

_____

_____

_____

_____

_____

_____

_____

_____

_____

_____

_____

_____

_____

_____

_____

My Prayer For Today

(This can be a personal prayer or reference a scripture)

Date: _____

_____

_____

_____

_____

_____

_____

_____

_____

_____

_____

_____

_____

_____

_____

_____

_____

_____

Date:_____

Today's Journal Entry

_____

_____

_____

_____

_____

_____

_____

_____

_____

_____

_____

_____

_____

_____

_____

_____

_____

_____

_____

_____

Date: _____

Identify the problem:

_____
_____
_____
_____
_____
_____
_____

Identify your thoughts and feelings related to the problem:

_____
_____
_____
_____
_____
_____
_____
_____
_____
_____
_____
_____

How can I challenge my thoughts and feelings related to the problem?

_____

_____

_____

_____

_____

1. Is there any proof or facts that support my thoughts and feelings? *(Only go by what you have heard verbatim from the source or seen directly.)* Have you addressed the situation to support your feelings?

Yes (Explain): _____

_____

_____

No (Explain): _____

_____

_____

2. What story, scenario, and or assumptions have I created in my head?

_____

_____

_____

_____

_____

_____

_____

3. After answering the previous two questions, share your new perspective, thoughts and feelings about the situation.

_____

_____

_____

_____

_____

_____

4. What is a realistic solution? Identify steps that help you move forward.

A. _____

_____

_____

B. _____

_____

_____

C. _____

_____

_____

D. _____

_____

_____

Daily Affirmations

I am:

_____

_____

_____

_____

_____

_____

_____

I will:

_____

_____

_____

_____

_____

_____

_____

I can:

_____

_____

_____

_____

_____

_____

Date: _____

Today's Goals

Today I will:

_____
_____
_____
_____
_____
_____
_____
_____
_____

Today I will not:

_____
_____
_____
_____
_____
_____
_____
_____
_____
_____

What I Am Grateful For

_____

_____

_____

_____

_____

_____

_____

_____

_____

_____

_____

_____

_____

_____

_____

_____

_____

_____

My Prayer For Today

(This can be a personal prayer or reference a scripture)

Date: _____

_____
_____
_____
_____
_____
_____
_____
_____
_____
_____
_____
_____
_____
_____
_____
_____
_____

Today's Journal Entry

_____
_____
_____
_____
_____
_____
_____
_____
_____
_____
_____
_____
_____
_____
_____
_____
_____
_____
_____
_____
_____

Date: _____

Identify the problem:

_____
_____
_____
_____
_____
_____
_____

Identify your thoughts and feelings related to the problem:

_____
_____
_____
_____
_____
_____
_____
_____
_____
_____
_____
_____
_____
_____

How can I challenge my thoughts and feelings related to the problem?

Date: _____

_____
_____
_____
_____
_____

1. Is there any proof or facts that support my thoughts and feelings ? *(Only go by what you have heard verbatim from the source or seen directly.)* Have you addressed the situation to support your feelings?

Yes (Explain): _____
_____
_____

No (Explain): _____
_____
_____

2. What story, scenario, and or assumptions have I created in my head?

_____
_____
_____
_____
_____
_____
_____
_____

3. After answering the previous two questions, share your new perspective, thoughts and feelings about the situation.

_____

_____

_____

_____

_____

_____

4. What is a realistic solution? Identify steps that help you move forward.

A._____

_____

_____

B._____

_____

_____

C._____

_____

_____

D._____

_____

_____

Daily Affirmations

I am:
_____

_____

_____

_____

_____

_____

_____

I will:
_____

_____

_____

_____

_____

_____

_____

I can:
_____

_____

_____

_____

_____

_____

Today's Goals

Today I will:

_____

_____

_____

_____

_____

_____

_____

_____

Today I will not:

_____

_____

_____

_____

_____

_____

_____

_____

What I Am Grateful For

_____

_____

_____

_____

_____

_____

_____

_____

_____

_____

_____

_____

_____

_____

_____

_____

_____

_____

_____

My Prayer For Today

(This can be a personal prayer or reference a scripture)

Date: _____

_____

_____

_____

_____

_____

_____

_____

_____

_____

_____

_____

_____

_____

_____

_____

_____

_____

_____

Date:_____

Today's Journal Entry

_____

_____

_____

_____

_____

_____

_____

_____

_____

_____

_____

_____

_____

_____

_____

_____

_____

_____

_____

Date: _____

Identify the problem:

_____

_____

_____

_____

_____

_____

Identify your thoughts and feelings related to the problem:

_____

_____

_____

_____

_____

_____

_____

_____

_____

_____

_____

How can I challenge my thoughts and feelings related to the problem?

_____

_____

_____

_____

_____

1. Is there any proof or facts that support my thoughts and feelings? *(Only go by what you have heard verbatim from the source or seen directly.)* Have you addressed the situation to support your feelings?

Yes (Explain): _____

_____

_____

No (Explain): _____

_____

_____

2. What story, scenario, and or assumptions have I created in my head?

_____

_____

_____

_____

_____

_____

_____

3. After answering the previous two questions, share your new perspective, thoughts and feelings about the situation.

_____

_____

_____

_____

_____

_____

4. What is a realistic solution? Identify steps that help you move forward.

A. _____

_____

_____

B. _____

_____

_____

C. _____

_____

_____

D. _____

_____

_____

Daily Affirmations

I am:
_____

_____

_____

_____

_____

_____

_____

I will:
_____

_____

_____

_____

_____

_____

_____

I can:
_____

_____

_____

_____

_____

_____

Today's Goals

Today I will:

_____

_____

_____

_____

_____

_____

_____

_____

Today I will not:

_____

_____

_____

_____

_____

_____

_____

_____

_____

What I Am Grateful For

_____

_____

_____

_____

_____

_____

_____

_____

_____

_____

_____

_____

_____

_____

_____

_____

_____

_____

My Prayer For Today

(This can be a personal prayer or reference a scripture)

Date: _____

_____

_____

_____

_____

_____

_____

_____

_____

_____

_____

_____

_____

_____

_____

_____

_____

Date:_____

Today's Journal Entry

_____

_____

_____

_____

_____

_____

_____

_____

_____

_____

_____

_____

_____

_____

_____

_____

_____

_____

_____

_____

Date: _____

Identify the problem:

_____

_____

_____

_____

_____

_____

_____

Identify your thoughts and feelings related to the problem:

_____

_____

_____

_____

_____

_____

_____

_____

_____

_____

_____

Date: _____

How can I challenge my thoughts and feelings related to the problem?

_____

_____

_____

_____

_____

1. Is there any proof or facts that support my thoughts and feelings ? *(Only go by what you have heard verbatim from the source or seen directly.)* Have you addressed the situation to support your feelings?

Yes (Explain): _____

_____

_____

No (Explain): _____

_____

_____

2. What story, scenario, and or assumptions have I created in my head?

_____

_____

_____

_____

_____

_____

_____

3. After answering the previous two questions, share your new perspective, thoughts and feelings about the situation.

_____

_____

_____

_____

_____

_____

4. What is a realistic solution? Identify steps that help you move forward.

A. _____

_____

_____

B. _____

_____

_____

C. _____

_____

_____

D. _____

_____

_____

Daily Affirmations

I am:

_____

_____

_____

_____

_____

_____

I will:

_____

_____

_____

_____

_____

_____

I can:

_____

_____

_____

_____

_____

Today's Goals

Today I will:

_____

_____

_____

_____

_____

_____

_____

_____

Today I will not:

_____

_____

_____

_____

_____

_____

_____

_____

What I Am Grateful For

_____

_____

_____

_____

_____

_____

_____

_____

_____

_____

_____

_____

_____

_____

_____

_____

_____

_____

_____

My Prayer For Today

(This can be a personal prayer or reference a scripture)

Date: _____

_____

_____

_____

_____

_____

_____

_____

_____

_____

_____

_____

_____

_____

_____

_____

_____

_____

Date:_____

Today's Journal Entry

_____

_____

_____

_____

_____

_____

_____

_____

_____

_____

_____

_____

_____

_____

_____

_____

_____

_____

_____

_____

_____

_____

Date: _____

Identify the problem:

_____

_____

_____

_____

_____

_____

_____

Identify your thoughts and feelings related to the problem:

_____

_____

_____

_____

_____

_____

_____

_____

_____

_____

_____

_____

How can I challenge my thoughts and feelings related to the problem?

_____

_____

_____

_____

_____

1. Is there any proof or facts that support my thoughts and feelings ? *(Only go by what you have heard verbatim from the source or seen directly.)* Have you addressed the situation to support your feelings?

Yes (Explain): _____

_____

_____

No (Explain): _____

_____

_____

2. What story, scenario, and or assumptions have I created in my head?

_____

_____

_____

_____

_____

_____

_____

3. After answering the previous two questions, share your new perspective, thoughts and feelings about the situation.

_____

_____

_____

_____

_____

_____

4. What is a realistic solution? Identify steps that help you move forward.

A. _____

_____

_____

B. _____

_____

_____

C. _____

_____

_____

D. _____

_____

_____

Daily Affirmations

I am:
_____

_____

_____

_____

_____

_____

I will:
_____

_____

_____

_____

_____

_____

I can:
_____

_____

_____

_____

_____

Today's Goals

Today I will:

_____

_____

_____

_____

_____

_____

_____

_____

_____

Today I will not:

_____

_____

_____

_____

_____

_____

_____

_____

_____

What I Am Grateful For

_____

_____

_____

_____

_____

_____

_____

_____

_____

_____

_____

_____

_____

_____

_____

_____

_____

_____

My Prayer For Today

(This can be a personal prayer or reference a scripture)

Date: _____

Date:_____

Today's Journal Entry

Date: _____

Identify the problem:

_____
_____
_____
_____
_____
_____
_____

Identify your thoughts and feelings related to the problem:

_____
_____
_____
_____
_____
_____
_____
_____
_____
_____
_____
_____

How can I challenge my thoughts and feelings related to the problem?

_____

_____

_____

_____

_____

1. Is there any proof or facts that support my thoughts and feelings? *(Only go by what you have heard verbatim from the source or seen directly.)* Have you addressed the situation to support your feelings?

Yes (Explain):

_____

_____

_____

No (Explain):

_____

_____

_____

2. What story, scenario, and or assumptions have I created in my head?

_____

_____

_____

_____

_____

_____

_____

_____

3. After answering the previous two questions, share your new perspective, thoughts and feelings about the situation.

_____

_____

_____

_____

_____

_____

4. What is a realistic solution? Identify steps that help you move forward.

A. _____

_____

_____

B. _____

_____

_____

C. _____

_____

_____

D. _____

_____

_____

Daily Affirmations

I am:

_____

_____

_____

_____

_____

_____

_____

I will:

_____

_____

_____

_____

_____

_____

_____

I can:

_____

_____

_____

_____

_____

_____

Today's Goals

Today I will:

_____

_____

_____

_____

_____

_____

_____

_____

_____

_____

Today I will not:

_____

_____

_____

_____

_____

_____

_____

_____

_____

_____

What I Am Grateful For

_____

_____

_____

_____

_____

_____

_____

_____

_____

_____

_____

_____

_____

_____

_____

_____

_____

_____

_____

_____

My Prayer For Today

Date: _____

_____

_____

_____

_____

_____

_____

_____

_____

_____

_____

_____

_____

_____

_____

_____

_____

Date: _____

Today's Journal Entry

_____

_____

_____

_____

_____

_____

_____

_____

_____

_____

_____

_____

_____

_____

_____

_____

_____

_____

_____

_____

_____

_____

Date: _____

Identify the problem:

_____

_____

_____

_____

_____

_____

_____

Identify your thoughts and feelings related to the problem:

_____

_____

_____

_____

_____

_____

_____

_____

_____

_____

_____

How can I challenge my thoughts and feelings related to the problem?

Date: _____

_____

_____

_____

_____

1. Is there any proof or facts that support my thoughts and feelings ? *(Only go by what you have heard verbatim from the source or seen directly.)* Have you addressed the situation to support your feelings?

Yes (Explain): _____

_____

_____

No (Explain): _____

_____

_____

2. What story, scenario, and or assumptions have I created in my head?

_____

_____

_____

_____

_____

_____

3. After answering the previous two questions, share your new perspective, thoughts and feelings about the situation.

_____

_____

_____

_____

_____

_____

4. What is a realistic solution? Identify steps that help you move forward.

A._____

_____

_____

B._____

_____

_____

C._____

_____

_____

D._____

_____

_____

Daily Affirmations

I am:

_____

_____

_____

_____

_____

_____

_____

I will:

_____

_____

_____

_____

_____

_____

_____

I can:

_____

_____

_____

_____

_____

_____

Date: _____

Today's Goals

Today I will:

_____
_____
_____
_____
_____
_____
_____
_____
_____

Today I will not:

_____
_____
_____
_____
_____
_____
_____
_____
_____
_____

What I Am Grateful For

_____

_____

_____

_____

_____

_____

_____

_____

_____

_____

_____

_____

_____

_____

_____

_____

_____

_____

My Prayer For Today

(This can be a personal prayer or reference a scripture)

Date: _____

_____

_____

_____

_____

_____

_____

_____

_____

_____

_____

_____

_____

_____

_____

_____

_____

Date:_____

Today's Journal Entry

Date: _____

Identify the problem:

_____
_____
_____
_____
_____
_____
_____

Identify your thoughts and feelings related to the problem:

_____
_____
_____
_____
_____
_____
_____
_____
_____
_____
_____
_____

How can I challenge my thoughts and feelings related to the problem?

_____

_____

_____

_____

_____

1. Is there any proof or facts that support my thoughts and feelings ? *(Only go by what you have heard verbatim from the source or seen directly.)* Have you addressed the situation to support your feelings?

Yes (Explain): _____

_____

_____

No (Explain): _____

_____

_____

2. What story, scenario, and or assumptions have I created in my head?

_____

_____

_____

_____

_____

_____

_____

3. After answering the previous two questions, share your new perspective, thoughts and feelings about the situation.

_____

_____

_____

_____

_____

_____

4. What is a realistic solution? Identify steps that help you move forward.

A. _____

_____

_____

B. _____

_____

_____

C. _____

_____

_____

D. _____

_____

_____

Daily Affirmations

I am:

_____

_____

_____

_____

_____

_____

_____

I will:

_____

_____

_____

_____

_____

_____

_____

I can:

_____

_____

_____

_____

_____

_____

Today's Goals

Today I will:

_____

_____

_____

_____

_____

_____

_____

_____

Today I will not:

_____

_____

_____

_____

_____

_____

_____

_____

What I Am Grateful For

_____

_____

_____

_____

_____

_____

_____

_____

_____

_____

_____

_____

_____

_____

_____

_____

_____

My Prayer For Today

(This can be a personal prayer or reference a scripture)

Date: _____

Date:_____

Today's Journal Entry

Date: _____

Identify the problem:

_____

_____

_____

_____

_____

_____

_____

Identify your thoughts and Feelings related to the problem:

_____

_____

_____

_____

_____

_____

_____

_____

_____

_____

_____

How can I challenge my thoughts and feelings related to the problem?

_____

_____

_____

_____

_____

_____

1. Is there any proof or facts that support my thoughts and feelings ? *(Only go by what you have heard verbatim from the source or seen directly.)* Have you addressed the situation to support your feelings?

Yes *(Explain)*: _____

_____

_____

No *(Explain)*: _____

_____

_____

2. What story, scenario, and or assumptions have I created in my head?

_____

_____

_____

_____

_____

_____

_____

_____

3. After answering the previous two questions, share your new perspective, thoughts and feelings about the situation.

_____

_____

_____

_____

_____

_____

4. What is a realistic solution? Identify steps that help you move forward.

A. _____

_____

_____

B. _____

_____

_____

C. _____

_____

_____

D. _____

_____

_____

Daily Affirmations

I am:

_____

_____

_____

_____

_____

_____

I will:

_____

_____

_____

_____

_____

_____

I can:

_____

_____

_____

_____

_____

Today's Goals

Today I will:

_____

_____

_____

_____

_____

_____

_____

_____

Today I will not:

_____

_____

_____

_____

_____

_____

_____

_____

_____

What I Am Grateful For

_____

_____

_____

_____

_____

_____

_____

_____

_____

_____

_____

_____

_____

_____

_____

_____

_____

My Prayer For Today

(This can be a personal prayer or reference a scripture)

Date: _____

_____

_____

_____

_____

_____

_____

_____

_____

_____

_____

_____

_____

_____

_____

_____

Date:_____

Today's Journal Entry

_____

_____

_____

_____

_____

_____

_____

_____

_____

_____

_____

_____

_____

_____

_____

_____

_____

_____

_____

_____

_____

_____

Date: _____

Identify the problem:

_____

_____

_____

_____

_____

_____

_____

Identify your thoughts and feelings related to the problem:

_____

_____

_____

_____

_____

_____

_____

_____

_____

_____

_____

_____

How can I challenge my thoughts and feelings related to the problem?

_____

_____

_____

_____

_____

1. Is there any proof or facts that support my thoughts and feelings ? (Only go by what you have heard verbatim from the source or seen directly.) Have you addressed the situation to support your feelings?

Yes (Explain):_____

_____

_____

No (Explain):_____

_____

_____

2. What story, scenario, and or assumptions have I created in my head?

_____

_____

_____

_____

_____

_____

_____

3. After answering the previous two questions, share your new perspective, thoughts and feelings about the situation.

_____

_____

_____

_____

_____

_____

4. What is a realistic solution? Identify steps that help you move forward.

A. _____

_____

_____

B. _____

_____

_____

C. _____

_____

_____

D. _____

_____

_____

Daily Affirmations

I am:

_____

_____

_____

_____

_____

_____

_____

I will:

_____

_____

_____

_____

_____

_____

_____

I can:

_____

_____

_____

_____

_____

Today's Goals

Today I will:

_____

_____

_____

_____

_____

_____

_____

_____

Today I will not:

_____

_____

_____

_____

_____

_____

_____

_____

What I Am Grateful For

_____

_____

_____

_____

_____

_____

_____

_____

_____

_____

_____

_____

_____

_____

_____

_____

_____

_____

_____

My Prayer For Today

(This can be a personal prayer or reference a scripture)

Date: _____

_____

_____

_____

_____

_____

_____

_____

_____

_____

_____

_____

_____

_____

_____

_____

Date:_____

Today's Journal Entry

Date: _____

Identify the problem:

_____

_____

_____

_____

_____

_____

_____

Identify your thoughts and feelings related to the problem:

_____

_____

_____

_____

_____

_____

_____

_____

_____

_____

_____

How can I challenge my thoughts and feelings related to the problem?

Date: _____

_____

_____

_____

_____

1. Is there any proof or facts that support my thoughts and feelings ? (Only go by what you have heard verbatim from the source or seen directly.) Have you addressed the situation to support your feelings?

Yes (Explain): _____

_____

_____

No (Explain): _____

_____

_____

2. What story, scenario, and or assumptions have I created in my head?

_____

_____

_____

_____

_____

_____

_____

3. After answering the previous two questions, share your new perspective, thoughts and feelings about the situation.

_____

_____

_____

_____

_____

_____

4. What is a realistic solution? Identify steps that help you move forward.

A. _____

_____

_____

B. _____

_____

_____

C. _____

_____

_____

D. _____

_____

_____

Daily Affirmations

I am:
_____

_____

_____

_____

_____

_____

_____

I will:
_____

_____

_____

_____

_____

_____

_____

I can:
_____

_____

_____

_____

_____

_____

Today's Goals

Today I will:

_____

_____

_____

_____

_____

_____

_____

_____

_____

Today I will not:

_____

_____

_____

_____

_____

_____

_____

_____

_____

What I Am Grateful For

_____

_____

_____

_____

_____

_____

_____

_____

_____

_____

_____

_____

_____

_____

_____

_____

_____

My Prayer For Today

(This can be a personal prayer or reference a scripture)

Date: _____

_____

_____

_____

_____

_____

_____

_____

_____

_____

_____

_____

_____

_____

_____

Date:_____

Today's Journal Entry

Date: _____

Identify the problem:

_____

_____

_____

_____

_____

_____

_____

Identify your thoughts and feelings related to the problem:

_____

_____

_____

_____

_____

_____

_____

_____

_____

_____

_____

_____

How can I challenge my thoughts and feelings related to the problem?

_____

_____

_____

_____

1. Is there any proof or facts that support my thoughts and feelings? *(Only go by what you have heard verbatim from the source or seen directly.)* Have you addressed the situation to support your feelings?

Yes (Explain): _____

_____

_____

_____

No (Explain): _____

_____

_____

2. What story, scenario, and or assumptions have I created in my head?

_____

_____

_____

_____

_____

_____

_____

3. After answering the previous two questions, share your new perspective, thoughts and feelings about the situation.

_____

_____

_____

_____

_____

_____

4. What is a realistic solution? Identify steps that help you move forward.

A. _____

_____

_____

B. _____

_____

_____

_____

C. _____

_____

_____

D. _____

_____

_____

Daily Affirmations

I am:

_____

_____

_____

_____

_____

_____

I will:

_____

_____

_____

_____

_____

_____

I can:

_____

_____

_____

_____

_____

_____

Today's Goals

Today I will:

_____

_____

_____

_____

_____

_____

_____

_____

_____

Today I will not:

_____

_____

_____

_____

_____

_____

_____

_____

_____

_____

What I Am Grateful For

_____

_____

_____

_____

_____

_____

_____

_____

_____

_____

_____

_____

_____

_____

_____

_____

_____

_____

My Prayer For Today

(This can be a personal prayer or reference a scripture)

Date: _____

Date:_____

Today's Journal Entry

_____

_____

_____

_____

_____

_____

_____

_____

_____

_____

_____

_____

_____

_____

_____

_____

_____

_____

_____

_____

_____

_____

Date: _____

Identify the problem:

_____
_____
_____
_____
_____
_____
_____

Identify your thoughts and Feelings related to the problem:

_____
_____
_____
_____
_____
_____
_____
_____
_____
_____
_____

How can I challenge my thoughts and Feelings related to the problem?

_____

_____

_____

_____

_____

1. Is there any proof or Facts that support my thoughts and Feelings ? *(Only go by what you have heard verbatim From the source or seen directly.)* Have you addressed the situation to support your Feelings?

Yes (Explain): _____

_____

_____

_____

No (Explain): _____

_____

_____

2. What story, scenario, and or assumptions have I created in my head?

_____

_____

_____

_____

_____

_____

_____

_____

3. After answering the previous two questions, share your new perspective, thoughts and feelings about the situation.

_____

_____

_____

_____

_____

_____

4. What is a realistic solution? Identify steps that help you move forward.

A. _____

_____

_____

B. _____

_____

_____

C. _____

_____

_____

D. _____

_____

_____

Daily Affirmations

I am:

_____

_____

_____

_____

_____

_____

I will:

_____

_____

_____

_____

_____

_____

I can:

_____

_____

_____

_____

_____

Today's Goals

Today I will:

_____
_____
_____
_____
_____
_____
_____
_____

Today I will not:

_____
_____
_____
_____
_____
_____
_____
_____
_____

What I Am Grateful For

_____

_____

_____

_____

_____

_____

_____

_____

_____

_____

_____

_____

_____

_____

_____

_____

_____

_____

_____

www.ingramcontent.com/pod-product-compliance
Lightning Source LLC
Chambersburg PA
CBHW020351130626
46549CB00006B/2254